The Chia Seed Weight Loss Diet

The natural and hunger free way to lose weight and feel good

Written by

Maggie Faye

Some people have a foolish way of not minding, or pretending not to mind, what they eat. For my part, I mind my belly very studiously, and very carefully; for I look upon it, that he who does not mind his belly will hardly mind anything else.
Samuel Johnson

Dedication

This book is dedicated to my three sons, Peter, Tony and David. They all have a sense of humor that keeps things in perspective when most needed, and are great fun to be around.

CONTENTS

INTRODUCTION

Imagine adding a nutrition loaded food to your diet that not only makes you feel healthier and more energetic, but also helps you lose weight without feeling hungry. It's a dieter's dream!

I don't know about you, but before I heard about chia seeds I had a constant battle with weight. Weight would creep on and I would put myself on a diet for several weeks. I tried many different diets and felt hungry, light headed and short tempered. Then when I stopped my diet, the weight would gradually creep back on again. Sound familiar?

Introducing the Chia seed. It is an ancient food from South America that has lately been making a comeback. The Mayan warriors, so it is said, could sustain themselves on a handful of the seeds per day plus water. They called it their running food because it gave them so much energy.

The chia seed is a nutritionally dense food. Gram for gram it gives you 8 times more omega 3s than salmon, 3 times more antioxidants than blueberries, a little more fiber than All Bran, 15 times more magnesium than broccoli. 6 times more calcium than whole milk and 3 times more iron than spinach. No wonder people feel good when they add chia seeds to their diet! All this, and yet chia seeds are low in calories and have a very low glycemic index, both very important considerations when eating for weight loss.

This book will show you how to use these wonderful little seeds as an aid to weight loss. It includes three methods to lose weight with chia seeds, easy ways to add the seeds to your diet for maximum weight loss effect, and a section on how to maintain your weight once you have reached your goal weight. There is also a section with easy chia seed recipes complete with the calorie count.

Once you have experienced the beneficial effects of eating chia seeds, you will want to keep them as a part of your diet, even after you have reached your goal weight.

I wrote this book from my own experience with chia seeds. While I was younger I would always diet before summer to lose the extra 10 to 20 pounds I had put on over winter.. But over the years it became more and more difficult to lose more than a few pounds when I dieted. Gradually my weight increased, and I reluctantly accepted that was a larger lady.

I still dieted but each year it became harder and harder to lose any weight. By the time I discovered chia seeds, I was carrying an extra 22 pounds over what is considered normal weight for my height. I felt chubby and unattractive. It may not have been a lot of extra weight , but it took me a lot of effort not to gain more. Dieting seemed to be just slowing down my weight gain.

When I first discovered chia seeds some 3 years ago, I was attracted to them for their health benefits. Imagine my surprise when, after a few weeks, I discovered I had lost a couple of pounds as well as feeling healthier, happier and more vibrant.

I began to experiment, by adding more chia seeds to my diet, up to about 3 or 4 tablespoons per day, I felt full, did not feel so hungry at meal times, and naturally served myself smaller meals. I felt no need for snacks between meals. I did not feel hungry, light headed or grumpy, as I usually did when dieting, but the weight kept gradually coming off. Needless to say, I was delighted!

Today I have lost my extra 22 pounds and kept it off for 2 years at least.

The only time I started to put weight back on was when I stayed for a month with my son who lives in another state. We had a great time, went out for meals a few times a week and often had fast food. I did not give my weight a thought and did not have chia seeds on hand. When I got back home, not only had I gained 7 pounds, but I felt sluggish.

It took me a few weeks, but I soon lost the extra weight I had put on and felt much more alive and healthy.

I have enjoyed writing this book and my wish is for you to enjoy it and benefit from the information inside by losing your extra weight and feeling healthy, happy and energetic.

Maggie Faye.

HOW WEIGHT LOSS WORKS

"Use or burn more energy than you intake and you will lose weight unless your body is the only one in the universe that defies the laws of physics. (Anon)

To lose weight successfully there are only two things you need to concentrate on.

The first is to burn more calories This is done by increasing your activity on a daily basis. The key here is the consistent, regular nature of the activities you choose. We will look more at easy ways to do this in the chapter on exercise. It's not as difficult as you think.
Increased activity on a regular basis makes losing weight easier and increases your muscle density. This is turn will tend to increase your metabolism which is important for keeping the weight off once you have lost it.

The added benefit of a little bit of extra activity is that it actually decreases your appetite. I'm not sure why but I have noticed this effect in my own weight loss journey.

The second is to take in fewer calories. This does not mean rigorous dieting or starvation. It is far better to concentrate on eating for health, choosing good nutrient dense foods (that is, foods that are full of vitamins and minerals) to satisfy you and also to look at eating smaller portions of this good food.

Chia seeds are dense in nutrients and low in calories, so are vegetables and fruit. The so-called superfoods, such as goji berries, seaweed, raw cacao, spirulina and others are also very high in nutrients and low in calories.

Starving yourself in order to lose weight is very unhealthy and not at all necessary. Starvation diets and extreme calorie restriction will make you feel tired, listless, unable or unmotivated to increase your activity. Even worse, you will lose muscle tissue and this will tend to decrease your metabolism over time. After such diets you are much more likely to put weight back on plus more if you try this method of weight loss.

Many people overeat because their bodies are actually starving even though they may be having more than enough calories. They may be overweight, but their bodies are lacking many of the essential vitamins and minerals. It saddens me, when I am in the supermarket and I see people stocking up on white bread, soft drinks, packaged, processed and refined foods and very little else. These people are invariably overweight.

The chia seed weight loss diet aims to give you a simple healthy way to lose weight, using the natural properties of chia seeds to increase your energy, keep you feeling full and give you sound nutrition, so you can take in fewer calories without feeling hungry.

HOW CHIA SEEDS HELP YOU LOSE WEIGHT

The little chia seed is only 74 calories per tablespoon. There is no magic ingredient in them that will make you lose weight, but by understanding their properties when adding them to your diet, you can use them as an effective aid to weight loss.

Chia seeds have the unique property of absorbing liquid.

They can absorb nine to twelve times their own weight of any liquid they are added to. This means they can be used to thicken soups, stews and gravies, thus extending the foods you eat and making you feel full more quickly without adding very many calories. Eating a chia pudding, chia gel or chia cookies will make you feel full and satisfied for a long time because of the seed's tendency to swell in size.

Chia seeds are high in nutrition

They provide a complete source of protein, are high in omega fats, minerals, B vitamins, calcium and antioxidants. For the amount of calories they contain, these seeds are extremely high in nutrients. Eating a healthy diet is one way to manage your weight, as you are then less likely to feel hungry. Eating foods that are low in nutrition can often lead to over eating as the body intuitively realizes that something is missing.

Chia seeds are digested slowly

Not only do chia seeds help you to feel full quickly, they also help you feel fuller for longer due to the way they digest slowly. When the seeds are added to liquid a gel forms around each seed. This gel slows down the digestion of the seeds. They digest at a slow and even rate, so blood sugar stays at a more even level. The high level of good fats and protein also aid in slowing down the rate at which they are absorbed. This tends to keep hunger at bay, making you less likely to look for between meal snacks.

Chia seeds are high in fiber

High fiber foods can help you feel full and they aid in regularity. You will notice your stomach feels and looks flatter after a few days of adding this food to your diet.

Chia seeds will increase your energy level

The high nutritional value of this food, plus its ability to release its energy providing nutrients slowly, means that you will feel more energetic for longer periods. Take advantage of this by increasing your activity level, exercising more or just walking more and burning more calories.

Understanding the properties of chia seeds and using them in your diet on a daily basis can help you eat less, eat a more nutritionally balanced diet and increase your energy and activity level. These are all things which can help you lose weight. In chapter 6 we will be looking at methods of adding chia seeds to your diet for the easiest and best ways to take advantage of the properties of chia seeds for weight loss, but first let's look at the health benefits of chia seeds.

CHIA SEED HEALTH BENEFITS

Let's take a moment to look at the health benefits of chia seeds. As we have seen chia seeds are a nutritionally dense food.

They have high amounts of:-

Omega 3 fatty acids.

Protein and this protein is complete, containing all essential amino acids.

Antioxidants

Vitamin Bs

Minerals

Yet they are low in calories and gluten free

Chia seeds are easy to digest. People who regularly eat chia seeds as part of their diet report the following benefits:-

Increased energy

Improved mood

More sustained energy levels

Improved concentration and clearer thinking

A decrease in aches and pains

A decrease in food cravings and less need to eat between meals

A feeling of well-being

Better regularity

Supple, smoother skin

Glossy hair and stronger nails

Research has shown chia seeds may be of benefit in improving cardiovascular health. This includes helping to reduce high blood pressure and high cholesterol levels. Research has also shown chia seeds can benefit brain and neurological functions, and arthritic conditions.

Chia seeds digest slowly. This tends to stabilize blood sugar which can be of help to people with type 2 diabetes or people who are pre-diabetic.
Chia seeds contain high levels of calcium, together with boron, which is of great benefit to bone health. For example, one tablespoon of chia seeds contain as much calcium as two glasses of milk.

Chia seeds can also prolong hydration and help retain electrolytes which makes them a great help to athletes, especially runners.

The high fiber of chia seeds, both soluble and insoluble, is a gentle way to maintain bowel health and promote regularity.

As you can see, chia seeds have great many health benefits and are a great addition to a healthy diet. The fact that they can assist in weight loss and weight management is an added bonus.

Now that you have a bit more knowledge of chia seeds and their properties, let's look at how to get started using chia seeds.

GETTING STARTED

Chia seeds have been a valuable food source for humans over many hundreds of years. They have recently been rediscovered and have rapidly gained favor as an addition to healthy eating in the modern world

While there are no known allergies to chia seeds, it is wise to be cautious when adding them to your diet if you have not eaten them before.

Start with one teaspoon of chia seeds on the first day. You can mix this in fruit juice, water, sprinkle them over cereal or just eat them raw from the spoon. Wait for one day, then have double the quantity. Wait another day and if you feel fine then try having a chia seed pudding (see recipe section) for breakfast. Wait another day. The vast majority of people experience only beneficial effects from adding chia seeds to their diet.

Caution – Chia seeds are known to have a blood thinning effect. For most people this can be beneficial, but if you are on blood thinning medication it is wise to seek medical advice before proceeding. In any case, if you are about to start a weight loss diet it is wise to seek medical advice.

A very few people report feeling bloated when adding chia seeds to their diet. If you feel this, then drink more water and it should settle down very quickly. This is most likely to happen if you have had a diet that is very low in fiber for a long time. The high fiber in chia seeds is very beneficial for the intestinal system and has a gentle cleansing effect on the bowel. You are soon likely to notice you have improved regularity and a flatter stomach. Drink plenty of water, 6 to 8 glasses a day - to aid this cleansing action.

Once you have introduced chia seeds to your diet and you are happy with the results, you are ready to start on the chia seeds weight loss diet.

THREE WAYS TO LOSE WEIGHT USING CHIA SEEDS

There are 3 methods of using chia seeds to lose weight.

The first of these I like to call the **Simple Method**. This involves taking a measured dose of chia seeds in liquid before each meal so that you feel full and want to eat less. It is an easy method, but can be a little boring. This method is for people who basically eat a healthy diet and only need to lose a few pounds in weight. It can also be a useful for people who are very busy and seldom have the time to prepare their own meals.

The second method is the **Meal Replacement Method**. For two meals a day, replace with a dish that is predominately made of chia seeds. It works well for people who are determined to lose weight in a short time and is suitable for those who want to lose any amount of weight. There is a selection of recipes to use for this method in the final chapter of this book.

The third method is the **Calorie Counting Method**. Counting calories is a little tedious, but many people, especially those who find it difficult to lose weight, often underestimate the number of calories they consume in a day. This method will help you to understand and apply ways to help with this problem.

The Simple Method

The simple method of weight loss using chia seeds makes use of the chia seeds properties to swell in liquid and to digest slowly. This makes you feel full and keeps you feeling full while the chia seeds digest.

Because the chia seeds contain a lot of healthy nutrients, it also gives you good nutrition which helps stop cravings for sweets and junk food.

This method is easy to follow and is suitable for people who basically eat a healthy diet and have only a few pounds they wish to lose. It's also suitable for busy people who have no time or desire for food preparation, or busy mums who have a family to feed and little time to prepare anything different for themselves.

Chia seeds are a healthy food and there are no official limits to the amount you can eat in a day, but for a weight loss diet I like to keep the amount of chia seeds consumed to between 2 and 4 tablespoons per day. There should be no need to have any more than that.

The Method

Immediately before each meal mix one tablespoon of chia seeds with half a glass of liquid and drink.

You can have your chia seeds in water, fruit juice or vegetable juice. If using fruit or vegetable juice, dilute with water, that is, one quarter of glass of juice plus one quarter of a glass of water. This is because juices have a lot of natural sugars which can be a hidden source of calories.

Remember, if you wait for more than a few seconds, the chia seeds will begin to absorb the liquid and swell. This will not make any difference to the diet, but you may need to eat it with a spoon.

Following this, drink one glass of water. This can be sipped gradually as you eat your meal or taken immediately after you have your chia seed drink.

You will feel full and not want to eat as much, so make sure the meal you eat is smaller than you would normally have. To remind you eat less at each meal, serve your meals on a smaller plate and eat more slowly. Don't hesitate to leave food on your plate when you feel full

Although this is a very simple method, it is very powerful, especially if you also take the trouble to eat wisely. You will lose weight more quickly and feel much healthier if you choose healthy meals. For example, choose salads instead of pasta, skip the rice, potatoes and bread. Choose fresh fruit for dessert or go without dessert entirely. In other words, load up on the fruit and vegetables which are low calorie and cut way down on the low nutrient empty calorie foods, such as white bread, sugary soft drinks, and desserts, pies and other pastries.

Do not eat between meals. If you do feel hungry between meals, this is an indication that you need to increase your serve of chia seeds. **You can increase this to one and a half tablespoon to a half glass of liquid if needed**.

If you have one tablespoon of chia seeds in your chia drink before meals, you will be having three tablespoons of chia seeds per day. If you increase this to one and a half tablespoons of chia seeds before each meal you will be having 4 and a half tablespoons of chia seeds per day.

Exercise

To increase your weight loss progress it is advisable to add half an hour of **extra e**xercise into your day. This can be as simple as a daily walk.

However, you will notice you have more energy when you add chia seeds to your diet on a daily basis. Don't be surprised if you spontaneously break into a little dance every now and then.

See more about boosting your weight loss with exercise in Chapter 10.

Advantages of the Simple Method

This method of using chia seeds for weight loss is simple and easy to follow. It uses no special recipes and there is no calorie counting. It's an easy diet to incorporate into a busy lifestyle. This method will work well for very many people.

Disadvantages of the Simple Method

Many people do not have any idea how many calories they are consuming each day. Many foods and meals have hidden calories. This is especially true if you eat out a lot or often have take-away meals. The simple method works best for people already eating a basically healthy diet with some knowledge of what foods can cause weight gain.

The Meal Replacement Method

This method of using chia seeds as for weight loss is more structured and more certain than the previous method. It gives more guidance on what foods to eat and it is ideal for those people who are a little uncertain of what foods can cause weight gain and those who have more than a few pounds of weight to lose. It also uses slightly more chia seeds per day than the simple method. Each replacement meal will generally use 1 to 2 tablespoons of chia seeds, giving you 2 to 4 tablespoons per day which will keep you feeling full, healthy and very energized.

This is my favorite method of losing weight with chia seeds. It gives you the pleasure and excitement of trying new dishes and it helps to re-educate your food choices. It gives you new, quick and easy meal options that you are likely to continue with after you have lost weight, which makes it easier for you to keep the weight off long term/

Chia seeds are a valuable food and can be used in many recipes. You will find directions for all the chia seed dishes suggested in this book in the recipes section, complete with the calorie count. There are more recipes on my website at www.chiaseedrecipes.com. Many of my readers have also contributed recipes and suggestions for using chia seeds.

Many commercial weight loss programs rely on the meal replacement model. By using chia seeds in this way you will be saving a lot of money, giving yourself more variety and looking after your nutritional health.

The Method

Replace two meals per day with a chia seed based meal. It is recommended that you replace breakfast and either lunch or dinner with a chia seed based meal.

The remaining meal should be a normal healthy meal with an emphasis on vegetables or salad and a good quality protein. Do not eat between meals and drink plenty of water.

Chia Seed Meal Replacement dishes

You will find the following recipes in the recipe section of this book. Each recipe has had the calories counted for your convenience and information.

Chia and fruit pudding - two Tablespoons chia seeds
Chia chocolate and raspberry pudding -two Tablespoons chia seeds
Fruit gel yogurt swirl -one and a half Tablespoons chia seeds
Smoothies -one Tablespoon chia seeds
Cauliflower chia soup with chia pan bread - two and a half Tablespoons chia seeds
Chia pan bread with cheese and tomato -two Tablespoon chia seeds
Chia pan bread with boiled or poached eggs -two Tablespoon chia seeds
Chia omelet with asparagus -one Tablespoon chia seeds
Chia pinole cookies with milk or orange juice -(4 cookies) two Tablespoons per serve
Chia pikelets -one Tablespoon chia seeds

Choose any two of the above for each day you are following the diet, then eat a normal healthy meal for the third meal of the day, whether it is lunch or dinner. For your third meal, make sure you have plenty of vegetables plus a small serving of some protein. **You can, if you wish, also have a chia drink, 1 tablespoon of chia seeds in a half glass of liquid plus a glass of plain water, before your normal meal**.

Have either a hot drink or a glass of water with or after each meal. The hot drink can be tea, coffee or green tea. Green tea is recommended because it has a beneficial effect on the metabolism and can assist with weight loss.

You are likely to find that you are less hungry than normal for this third meal. If so, serve yourself less. Don't be afraid to leave food on your plate The important thing is to let your body tell you how much to eat.

The high nutritional value of chia seeds will make you less likely to have food cravings or feel hungry even if you are eating less than usual. The ability of the chia seeds to absorb liquid and digest slowly will have you quickly feeling satisfied and satisfied for longer. Remember to drink plenty of water throughout the day and refrain from eating between meals.

Exercise

As with the Simple Method, it will be beneficial to boost your weight loss with added exercise. It is only necessary to add half an hour of extra activity per day to increase your metabolism and to make a difference to your weight loss progress.

Advantages of the Meal Replacement method

You are more in control with this method and consequently more certain to lose the weight you want.

Disadvantages of the Meal Replacement method

Although the recipes are generally very quick and easy, there is more work, organization and planning with this method.

The Calorie Counting Method

Calorie counting should not be necessary if you follow the meal replacement method as outlined in the previous chapter. However, I have included this method because some people underestimate how many calories they eat in a day. Other people feel more secure if they know how many calories they should eat in a day if they want to lose weight.

It is important to keep a food diary and put down everything you eat with the calorie counting method. This is tedious and time consuming, but you will know exactly how many calories you are consuming each day with this method. If you decide to follow this method, there are several online websites where you can keep a food diary and calculate the amount of calories you consume each day. A good one can be found at fitday.com. It will calculate your ideal calorie intake depending on your activity level, age and gender and has calorie counts for thousands of foods

Know your ideal calorie consumption

The calories you need to maintain an ideal body weight depends on your height, age, gender and activity level. The average, moderately active younger woman needs around 2,000 to 2,200 calories per day to maintain body weight. The average, moderately active younger man needs around 2,600 to 2, 800 calories per day.

For every decade over 30 you are, subtract 100 calories per day from the above numbers.

If you are more used to kilojoules, 100 calories converts to 420 Kj and 2,000 calories converts to 8,400 Kj

How many calories are needed for weight loss

In order to lose weight you need to take in fewer calories than you need to maintain your existing body weight. Exercising can help you burn more calories and it is advisable to add half an hour of increased activity to aid in weight loss.

It is generally recommended to reduce your calorie intake by 400 to 800 calories per day to lose weight in a consistent manner. It is not recommended to go below 1,300 calories for a woman or 1,800 calories for a man. If in doubt this is something you should discuss with your doctor.

Above all do not go below the lower recommended limits of calorie intake for weight loss. If you do, your body can go into starvation mode and it will retain the excess weight you have. A prolonged starvation level diet can reduce your metabolism which will make it even harder for you to lose weight.

The Method

Follow the meal replacement diet. For your convenience all the meal replacement recipes have had the calories counted. Keep a food diary, preferably online at a site like fitday.com and record your calorie consumption. You will be able to enter your weight, age and activity level to get your recommended calorie consumption on the website.

Exercise

Increase your activity level by exercising for half an hour each day. A half hour walk is a simple way to do this. See Chapter 10 for more on exercising.

Advantages of the Calorie Counting Method

You are adopting a sure, proven, scientific way of weight loss by using this method, and you will learn a lot about the calorie values of the foods you eat. This can help you choose better foods to eat and make it easier to maintain your ideal weight for life.

Disadvantages of the Calorie Counting Method

It takes time and it can be tedious keeping count of the calories you eat each day.

ADDING EXERCISE

To boost your weight loss while dieting it is recommended to add at least a half hour of extra activity to your day. This can be as simple as adding half an hour of walking to your day. This half hour of extra activity can be done in short bursts of activity, such as 3 lots of 10 minutes.

This extra activity will help you to burn more calories and make your weight loss happen faster. It will also mean you build more muscle tissue which can increase your metabolism, making it easier for you to maintain your ideal weight.

By adding chia seeds to your diet you will feel more energetic and feel as though you want to be more active.

Simple and fun ways of adding this extra activity to your day

Walk a dog/ your own or someone else's
Play outside with the kids
Take the stairs wherever possible instead of using an elevator
Take up bike riding again\
Put on some music and dance for 10 minutes to half an hour
Offer to mow someone's lawn
Jump rope
Run or march on the spot
Pretend to be a conductor to some fast music this is surprisingly effective

The key thing is to do something on a regular basis. For example, make it a habit to park the car some distance away from where you want to go. The extra activity does add up over the course of a day.

One very effective way to exercise is to use a pedometer and aim to walk 10,000 steps each day. That is quite a bit of walking and it encourages you to get up and move around more. At the end of the day if you have not reached your goal of 10,000 steps, then you can march on the spot while watching television, doing the washing up or supervising the kid's homework.

Of course if you want to do more, you can join a gym or take up a new sport, and if you have exercise equipment, make sure you use it instead of storing it conveniently under the bed. Adding chia seeds to your diet will give you extra, sustained energy which may motivate you to take up your favorite sport again.

FOODS TO AVOID

Going on a weight loss diet should not be an exercise in deprivation and starvation. It should be looked at as an education in healthy eating. People who eat a healthy diet tend to have fewer issues around weight gain.

One of the main reasons people put on weight is because they eat too many of the wrong foods. Foods that are likely to make you gain weight are the ones that are high in calories and low in essential nutrients.

If you are eating a lot of foods that are low in nutrients, then even if you have enough calories for your body, you will feel listless and unsatisfied. Your body will instinctively know that you have not had enough nutrients (protein, vitamins, healthy fats and minerals) and you will more than likely suffer from food cravings and want to overeat to compensate for the lack of good nutrition.

It is no coincidence that the rate of obesity has gone up steadily in correlation with the increase in the consumption of sugar over the past 50 years in western countries. Refined flours are almost as bad, because they digest quickly, have few nutrients, and leave your body feeling unsatisfied.

The following is a list of foods to avoid if you want to lose weight.

All sugary drinks including sodas, diet sodas, iced coffees, bottled iced teas and alcohol. Substitute these drinks with water. If you must have sodas, don't substitute with zero calorie drinks. Not only are they sweetened with harmful chemicals, but research has shown they are ineffective in weight loss because they do not satisfy the body's perceived need for real sugar.

Try my healthy alternative. Take one bottle of sparkling mineral water. Pour out 1 glass of the contents to prevent it frothing over. Add a squeeze of lemon juice to your bottle of mineral water. Its tangy and has bubbles. I like it just like that, but if you need sweetness, add in a little stevia – a natural sweetener with no calories that is derived from the leaf of the stevia plant. Carefully pour back the contents of the glass, and you have a healthy no-cal lemonade. Using a funnel to add the stevia and lemon juice does help.

Low nutrition snacks including popcorn, candy, potato chips, cookies, cakes and ice-cream.

Salty foods- too much salt can make your body hang onto water weight

Fried foods, especially deep fried foods. Use non-stick pans or spray on oils instead
.

Fast foods, they are usually deep fried or otherwise high in unhealthy fats making them high in calories.

Added sugars, including corn syrup and fructose. These are just empty calories and mess with your blood sugar levels.

Processed foods much of the good nutrition has often been taken out and replaced with high levels of sugar, fats and chemical preservatives.

Pies and pastries - pastries are made mostly of white flour and fats, have little nutrition and are high in calories.

Jams and preserves – very high in sugar.

While on a weight loss diet it is best if you stick to whole, natural foods. Have plenty of vegetables, some good quality protein (eggs, low fat meat, chicken, beans, lentils or a small portion of cheese) and fresh fruit. Limit the amount of bread and pasta you consume and go for whole grain versions for better nutrition. Fruit juices should also be limited as they are high in sugars. Fruit juices are best consumed with chia seeds, such as a fruit juice gel or a smoothie to give a more sustained release of energy.

I have found that adding chia seeds to your diet reduces blood sugar highs and lows, making you far less likely to want the types of food listed above.

TROUBLESHOOTING, QUESTIONS AND ANSWERS

On the chia seed weight loss diet you should lose weight steadily, generally at 1 to 2 pounds a week, sometimes more, especially if you choose to adopt the chia seed meal replacement model and you are exercising on a regular basis.

If after a week or two you have not started to lose weight, the most likely thing is that you have underestimated the amount of food you are eating or you are eating too many high calorie foods. The best way round this is to keep a food diary. Make a promise to yourself that you will not eat anything unless you have written it down first!

Take another look at the list of foods to avoid and remind yourself not to eat food from this list. Your mind and body will thank you for this and the pounds will gradually melt away.

Keeping a food diary will ensure you do not suffer from food amnesia. It is easy to forget some of the foods we have eaten during the day, especially if we are busy doing other things. Did you remember to include the cappuccino you had with lunch (84 calories) or the glass of white wine with dinner (122 calories). Don't allow yourself to be tempted to eat between meals. Keeping a food diary will soon make you stop and think before you take a bite of anything, especially between meals.

Remember to eat smaller meals than usual if you are using the simple method of weight loss. To help with this serve your meals on a smaller plate, and load it up with low calorie vegetables or salads before putting anything else on the plate. Or consider moving on to the meal replacement method for more certain results.

Another type of food amnesia trap can occur if you cook for other people and have to taste the food before serving. Each taste could amount to 25 calories, not much, but it can add up over the course of a day to 100, 150 or even 200 calories. Keep this type of eating to a minimum. Take only the smallest possible taste and only taste when absolutely necessary.

Look again at the amount of exercise you are doing. Half an hour of exercising, walking, dancing, bike riding does help to shift the pounds. With chia seeds added to your diet you should be feeling more energetic and more motivated to keep moving.

An occasional problem with adding chia seeds to your diet can be constipation. Most people find the gentle cleansing properties of high fiber chia seeds keeps them regular and feeling very comfortable in the abdominal region. If you are experiencing any constipation, it's more than likely because you are not drinking enough water, so increase the amount of water you have per day and it should not be a problem. Make sure you are drinking the recommended 8 glasses of water per day.

The following is a list of typical questions and answers from my chia seed recipes site which I hope you will find useful.

Which seeds should I use, black or white?

You can use either. There is little difference between black and white seeds. I prefer to use the white seeds if I want chia seeds to blend into a dish I am making, such as a milk pudding, but this is by no means necessary. Nutritionally the black seeds have slightly more antioxidants.

Is it necessary to grind the chia seeds to get the full nutritional value from them?
No. Unlike flax seeds which are difficult to digest fully in their whole form, chia seeds are fully digested when eaten whole.

I was making a chia gel and the chia seeds clumped together in a hard mass on the bottom of my bowl. How do I prevent this?
You need to whisk them into the liquid for about 20 seconds, then give the mixture a stir every 30 seconds or so until the gel starts to form. Once the mixture has gelled, the seeds will not separate out. The gel will form within 5 to 10 minutes.

Do I need to store my chia seeds in the fridge? How long will they keep?
Chia seeds are very high in antioxidants and will keep well for at least 2 years stored in a kitchen cupboard or pantry.

Do I need to soak chia seeds before using them?
When adding whole chia seeds to liquids, such as puddings, gels, smoothies soups or casseroles there is no need to soak them. They will soften and swell in the liquid used in your recipe. When adding chia seeds to dry mixtures such as cookies, muffins or bread mixes, it is best to use ground chia seeds and again, there is no need to soak. Some people like to sprinkle dry seeds over salads. This gives a crunchy texture which some people like.

What is the difference between milled chia seeds and ground chia seeds?
There is no difference. When I first started using chia seeds, I could only obtain whole chia seeds and I ground them in a coffee grinder when I wanted to make cookies or bread. Now milled chia is readily available.

How do I know if my seeds are good quality?
Always buy recognized good quality brands for a start. Quality chia seeds should be either black or a greyish white. There will be a few white seeds in a pack of black chia seeds and a few black ones in the white chia seeds. If your seeds are brown, they are low quality, immature seeds and may even contain some weed seeds among them. Often they will not even gel properly.

MAINTENANCE

What do you do once you have reached your goal weight? If you return to the way you were eating before you reached your goal weight, then you will end up putting weight on until you are right back where you started.

The best way to prevent this is to continue eating mostly good whole foods and keep chia seeds as a regular part of your daily food intake. I like to have chia seeds regularly, one to two tablespoons per day at least 5 days a week. You will feel healthier and more energetic if you change your old eating, habits, adopt a more healthy diet and keep chia seeds on your menu as part of your regular diet.

Remember to weight yourself at least on a weekly or fortnightly basis. It is far easier to correct a 2 to 5 pound weight gain than a 20 pound weight gain. Your weight tends to fluctuate during the day so weighing yourself at the same time each day gives you a more accurate measure.

I have made it a habit to weigh myself each morning. My weight is steady now. I can't begin to tell you how satisfying it is to see that same figure showing each morning.

If you have gained a few extra pounds, then it's simple to go back on one of the chia seed diets for a week or two until you are once again back at your ideal weight. However, I believe that if you regularly take one or two tablespoons of chia seeds daily you will seldom need to do that.

Chia seeds have helped me to eat less and still feel full. It's as though they have reset my appetite. They have also helped me to choose foods more wisely. I no longer have the food cravings I used to have. I firmly believe food cravings are an indication of poor nutrition. Of course, I still have the occasional chocolate bar, cheese cake or pastry, but I am not drawn to them as I used to be. The occasions when I do have such foods are just naturally becoming fewer and fewer.

Maintaining your ideal weight with chia seeds is easy. It can easily be a simple no fuss smoothie, chia fruit gel with yogurt, or a chia seed pudding for breakfast. Starting the day in this way will give you good nutrition, give you sustained energy, and make you feel less like indulging in the wrong foods during the day.

If you have a lot of weight to lose it's a good idea to take a break every 4 weeks or so and go on to the maintenance level for a week. Congratulate yourself if you are eating less than before and making better food choices. Keep going at 4 weeks on the chia seed weight loss diet, one week on maintenance until you have reached your desired weight.

CHIA SEED MEAL REPLACEMENT RECIPES

The following recipes have all had the calories estimated. The calories for each recipe are generally between 300 and 400 calories. Two of these replacement meals will give approximately 700 to 800 calories, combined allowing you to have a good sized third meal for the day and still lose weight.

Don't feel you have to be restricted to these recipes only. If you have your own favorite ways to enjoy chia seeds, then feel free to have your chia seeds however you enjoy them.

I have kept these recipes simple, quick and easy to make, but if you are in a situation where you have not had the time to prepare one of them, don't hesitate to have a tablespoon of chia seeds in water before you eat your next meal as outlined in the simple method. The aim is to make weight loss easy, not a chore.

Chia cauliflower soup

This makes 2 serves. It's a quick and easy soup to make. You can either save the extra serve for the following day or share it with someone.

Ingredients

half a cauliflower cut into small pieces

one small onion

2 heaped teaspoons of good quality stock powder **or** 2

stock cubes **or** 2 cups of stock

sea salt to taste if required

1 tablespoon of freshly ground chia seeds

2 cups of water (omit if you have used liquid stock)

Method

Chop the onion and put into a pot with the small cauliflower pieces and the vegetable stock powder.

Add 2 cups water and bring to the boil. Simmer for about 15 minutes.

Take out half the mixture and blend with the ground chia seeds, Return this mixture to the pot and stir through, The result a lovely thick, creamy cauliflower soup. If you find this soup is a little too thick for your liking, you can add a little water. Serve with a lightly buttered chia pan bread bun and a refreshing green salad with a squeeze of lemon juice for dressing (optional).

Reminder:- The serve of chia pan bread should be half of the amount given in the recipe for chia pan bread. That recipe makes 2 flat hamburger sized buns.

Calories for 1 serve of soup 1 buttered chia bun and green salad is 379

Chia Seed Omelet with Asparagus

Ingredients for one serve

I tablespoon chia seeds

2 tablespoons water

2 eggs

4 asparagus spears

Method

Put 1 tablespoon chia seeds, 2 tablespoons of water and the eggs in a bowl, whisk together and let the mixture stand for 10 to 20 minutes. Stir this mixture every 30 seconds or so to prevent the seeds clumping together.
Steam 4 asparagus spears.
Melt a small knob of butter in a non-stick pan
Whisk egg and chia seed mix again to prevent seeds settling out.
Pour into pan and cook gently until top is set. Using a lid will help the top set faster
Season to taste, put asparagus spears in center, fold the omelet over and serve.

The above recipe uses whole chia seeds, but if you prefer you can grind the seeds before adding the other ingredients, or use store bought milled chia seeds. Alternatively, you can blend the mixture before cooking which gives a similar effect to using ground chia seeds.

275 calories

Chia banana pikelets

This recipe makes 8 pikelets which is enough for 2 people or 2 serves

Ingredients
1/2 cup of plain flour

2 tablespoons ground chia seeds (or use store bought milled chia seeds)

1and a half teaspoons baking powder

60g plain yogurt (4 T or quarter cup)

half mashed banana

half teaspoon vanilla extract

2 eggs, separated

1 banana for topping

Two teaspoons of honey

Method
Grind chia seeds in a coffee grinder or use milled chia seeds
Combine flour, ground chia seeds and baking powder.

In a separate bowl, mix yogurt, egg yolks, mashed banana and a splash of water(about two teaspoons). Mix into batter. You may need to use a little extra water if the mixture is a little stiff.

Beat egg white in an electric blender until soft peaks form.
Mix the egg whites into the batter

Heat a little olive oil in a non stick pan.
Drop tablespoons spoons of batter into pan when hot
Cook gently, turning when light brown. Takes about
5minutes each side. Makes 8 pikelets

Serve warm with a drizzle of honey over the top and a

small sliced banana.

**Calories 350 per serve of 4 with half a small banana per
serve**

Chia pan bread

Makes two flat hamburger sized buns which can be sliced in half to make the recommended dishes here.

Ingredients

4 Tablespoons ground chia seed (grind 4 T chia seeds or buy milled chia seeds)

4 Tablespoons plain flour of choice - quinoa flour is good

1 teaspoon of baking powder

1 egg

Half a small onion/or half a small zucchini/or same quantity grated carrot

Method

Take ground chia seeds and place in a bowl with the flour and baking powder.
Mix well.
Blend the egg with the onion or other vegetable of choice until smooth.
Mix the egg mixture with the dry ingredients.
Turn onto a floured board, kneed until all ingredients are combined well and flatten out until quite thin.
Divide into two and shape into two hamburger sized buns
Oil a heavy based fry-pan and cook them for a few minutes or either side preferably with the lid on as this will help the bread to rise. Slice through when cool and add toppings.

329 calories for the whole pan bread recipe. 165 calories per bun

Chia Pan Bread Meal Replacements

Chia Pan Bread with cheese and tomato

Take one chia pan bread bun and slice carefully in two
On each half add sliced tomato and a good slice of cheese
Grill until cheese starts to melt.

This dish has 352 calories

Chia Pan bread with poached or boiled eggs

Take one chia pan bread bun and slice carefully in half
Lightly butter each half
Add a poached egg on each half
or
Add sliced boiled eggs to each half using two eggs

This dish has 340 calories

Chia Pinole cookies

The ingredients below are for 16 cookies. I like to use quinoa flour but any good quality flour will do. I have used potato flour, oatmeal finely ground, almond flour as well as wheat flour

Ingredients

8 Tablespoons of ground chia seeds

2 teaspoons of cinnamon

4 Tablespoons of flour (quinoa flour if available)

2 Tablespoons of rolled oats

2 Tablespoons of chopped dried fruit

4 Tablespoons of honey

2 eggs

Method

Grind the chia seeds in a blender or coffee grinder or buy milled chia seeds
Add the cinnamon, flour and rolled oats
Toast these ingredients carefully in a frying pan until very slightly brown
Allow to cool
Add the dried fruit

Blend the eggs and honey in a blender and stir into the dry ingredients, adding a little water if needed.
Spoon the mixture onto an oiled or non-stick baking tray and flatten them out
Bake in a moderate oven for about 15 minutes or until browned.

Each cookie is 56 calories 4 cookies can be used as a meal replacement, giving 224 calories

When you have 4 chia pinole cookies as a meal replacement, have with either a cup of unsweetened orange juice adding **112 calories (total 336 calories) or a cup of milk adding 122 calories (total 346 calories)**

Two chia pinole cookies with a cup of unsweetened green tea is an effective between meal snack at 112 calories if absolutely needed.

These smoothies are an ideal and easy way to get a daily serve of chia seeds whether or not you are on a weight loss diet. I like to soak the seeds for 10 minutes or more in the juice to soften them, remembering to whisk the mixture a few times to prevent clumping and allow the seeds to soften and swell. This makes the smoothies smoother. If any of the smoothies are a little too thick for your liking, just add a little water. I prefer not to add any sweeteners to the smoothies, but a little stevia or honey can be added if you like. Drink your smoothie immediately as it will continue to thicken if you let it stand.

Apple Banana Smoothie

Ingredients

half a medium banana

1and a half cups of apple juice

1 tablespoon chia seeds

1 to 2 teaspoons honey (optional)

Method

Soak the chia seeds in the apple juice for 10 minutes to soften them.

Stir or whisk the mixture a few times to stop the seeds clumping together.

Slice the banana into the juice and seed mixture add honey (if required)

Blend until smooth.

Calories 293 calories without honey, 327 with honey

Orange Mango Cream Smoothie

Ingredients

1and a half cups of good quality unsweetened orange juice

Half cup of ripe mango

Half a banana

2 Tablespoons of plain yogurt

1 tablespoon of chia seeds

1 or two teaspoons of honey (optional)

Method

Soak the chia seeds in the orange juice for 10 minute to let
them swell and soften

Put all ingredients in your blender

Blend well until creamy.

Enjoy!

Calories 375 calories without honey, 409 with honey

Merry Berry Smoothie simple, quick and low cal

Ingredients

1 and a half cups of apple juice

1 cup of mixed berries frozen or fresh

1 tablespoon of chia seeds

2 teaspoons of honey (optional)

Method

Soak the chia seeds in the apple juice for 10 minutes or so.

Blend all ingredients together until smooth

Calories 296 without honey, 330 calories with honey

Pina colada chia smoothie

Ingredients

Half banana

Half an orange, seeded, peeled and chopped

Half a cup pineapple cut small

a couple of slices of ripe mango,

Half cup coconut milk

Half cup water

1 Tablespoon chia seeds

2 teaspoons of honey (optional)

Method

Soak the seeds in the water/coconut milk mixture for at least 10 minutes stirring occasionally to prevent the seeds from clumping together

Blend all the ingredients together until smooth

Enjoy!

This smoothie has quite a lot of calories, mainly from the coconut milk, but it will keep you full and satisfied for a long time.

Calories 461 calories without honey, 495 calories with honey

Fruit gel yogurt swirl

This is a refreshing, filling and nourishing summer breakfast, and very quick and easy to make.

Ingredients

1 serve of plain unsweetened yogurt (about a cupful)

1 and a half tablespoons of chia seeds

Half a cup of good quality unsweetened fruit juice

Cranberry, pomegranate, mixed berry, cloudy apple, apple and mango, orange and mango and apricot all taste great. Of course, you can also juice your own fruit.

Method

Mix the chia seeds into the juice and leave for 10 to 15 minutes to form a gel. Whisk the mixture a couple of times during this time to prevent the seeds clumping together. Put the yogurt into a bowl, pour the fruit juice gel over the top then swirl the gel through a couple of times.

It looks and tastes much nicer if you can see the two toned effect, but some people like to mix the gel and yogurt together more thoroughly. Experiment to see which way you prefer yours.

This recipe gives 321 calories per serve

Chia puddings

When making chia seed puddings or gels, remember to whisk the seeds through the liquid thoroughly, let stand for 30 seconds to a minute then whisk again. This stops the seeds clumping together before they have fully expanded. Check a few times while the pudding is standing as you may need to whisk the mixture again.

You can make chia puddings from any type of milk, such as almond milk, coconut milk, rice milk, oat milk, goat milk as well as cow's milk. Let your own taste and imagination be your guide.

The following chia pudding recipes are an example of some of the ways I have used chia seeds to make puddings. I find they make a very quick and easy breakfast or even lunch,

Chia Banana Pudding

You can add any fresh fruit to this dish if you don't like banana. Calories would probably be a little less. It can also be made with cold milk if you prefer.

Ingredients for one serve

2 tablespoons of Chia seeds

I cup of milk

sea salt to taste

2 teaspoons of honey

1 small banana

Method

Heat the milk but do not boil
Whisk the chia seeds into the hot milk and let stand for 10/15 minutes to make a gel
Whisk the mixture a few times within this time to prevent the seeds clumping together
Reheat the mixture after standing if required
slice banana over the top and drizzle with honey
2 tablespoons makes quite a thick mixture. Add a little more milk if you want it thinner.

Calories 390 with 2 Tablespoons chia seeds

Ideas
Use ground chia seeds instead of whole seeds. This is very warming in cold weather. The seeds can be ground in a

blender or coffee grinder or you can buy ready-milled chia seeds.

This can also be made with cold milk which is very refreshing in warm weather. Just add the chia seeds to cold milk and let it stand for around 15 minutes to let the chia seeds swell and thicken the mixture. Remember to stir or whisk the mixture a few times during this time.

Chocolate Raspberry Chia seed pudding

Use cold milk for this recipe and make a basic chia pudding as above.

Sprinkle 1 Tablespoon of choc chips or 1 Tablespoon of chocolate syrup over the chia and milk mix once it has gelled. Add half a cup of fresh raspberries.

Calories 400 if using 2 Tablespoons of chia seeds

ABOUT THE AUTHOR – Maggie Faye

I was born in Australia, and like many Australians, I have lived, worked and travelled to many overseas destinations, including Malaysia, Indonesia, Singapore, South Africa, France and the United Kingdom.

This has enabled me to indulge in my great passion for interesting food. I will sample and probably enjoy any interesting local dish on offer. I have fond memories of Scottish Haggis, Malaysian Laksa, Singapore drunken prawns and South African peri-peri chicken to name a few.

My interest in chia seeds began around 3 years ago. I love finding new ways to prepare and use them, and they have had such a beneficial effect on my health that they will always be a staple food in my pantry.

I invite all my readers to visit me at my site, http://www.chiaseedrecipes.com
We have an active comments area, where people share their recipes and success stories. Many people have queries about chia seeds and I am always happy to answer them. I look forward to hearing your success stories and new ways to use chia seeds.

INDEX OF RECIPES

Made in the USA
Lexington, KY
29 November 2013